Sugar Free Cookbook

Simple and Delicious Recipes For An Easy Start Into A Sugar-Free Life

Alison Bojarska

Table of the Contents:

Introduction

Wrong food makes you sick

Many of our staple foods make you sick. This is due to the frequent consumption and also to your attitude towards life. We take our time for everything, the nice movie night, the chat at the bar and the waiting at the supermarket checkout. Only our daily food has to be done quickly and easily. Mostly without questioning, the main thing is that the annoying feeling of hunger is stopped. Low carb takes a holistic approach. Without a corset and your own diet. Eat yourself healthy without getting round.

Our food is therefore subject to a modular system. Trans fats, lots of carbohydrates and sugar are only partially subject to our nutrition plan. Our organism needs vitamins, minerals, trace elements, everything so that we can stay healthy and fit. Especially the sugar-free, with low carb, really starts here. Without stressing, but with a lot of sensitivity in the selection of ingredients. Bans lead to renunciation and renunciation desires the forbidden. A simple rule that says eat healthy without going hungry. Because hunger is the greatest enemy and has been proven to make you fat. As a result, low carb is a tried and tested nutritional system for people like you and me.

What is sugar

Sugar is used both as a luxury food and as a food. Sugar used to be very special and few people could afford it. It is now no longer expensive and is available everywhere. In recent years, however, sugar has lost its popularity and has come under increasing criticism. It is unhealthy, makes you fat and is harmful to your teeth. Sugar is basically just a carbohydrate and serves as a source of energy. It is mainly obtained from plants. From a chemical point of view, the common sugar is a disaccharide, also known as a disaccharide. It is made up of monosaccharides (simple sugars) and fructose.

Since sugar is a carbohydrate, it plays an important role in the diet, because over 50% of the energy the human body needs should come from carbohydrates. The brain already uses 140 g of glucose every day. That's as much as 14 tablespoons of sugar. Pure sugar quickly travels into the blood and from there to the brain. So if energy is needed very quickly, as is sometimes the case with exercise, then sugar, especially grape sugar, is very suitable. However, this is digested again very quickly and the feeling of hunger comes back after a short time. Since sugar contains almost no nutrients, it is also referred to as "empty calories". Carbohydrates are also found in potatoes, pasta and flour. However, the intestines first have to break them down, so that the energy from these foods is available longer.

How is sugar made?
The effects of sugar in the body

When sugar is absorbed, the blood sugar level rises immediately and insulin is released because the body compensates for the amount of sugar it has absorbed. Insulin is produced in the pancreas and is one of the hormones. It is responsible for breaking the sugar out of the blood and passing it on to other organs. Often times one feels good and happy after a piece of chocolate. This is also related to the insulin, because the hormone also causes serotonin to be formed in the body. This hormone is also known as the happiness hormone because it lifts your spirits.

Sugar free diets

Doing without sugar is not as easy as it sounds at first, because now almost all foods contain sweetness. For this reason, sugar should not be completely eliminated overnight. It is advisable to do without it gradually. Morning coffee, for example, can be sweetened with just one lump of sugar instead of the usual two. But unfortunately there are also many types of sugar that are hidden in products and foods and are not immediately recognizable. Even the breakfast cereals in the morning, which are advertised as "healthy", often contain more than 10% sugar. Sausage and ready meals are often mixed with quite a bit of sugar. It is therefore important to pay attention to the ingredients and to prepare the meals yourself if possible.

1. As soon as you decide to remove sugar from your list of ingredients, you start to read the ingredients of the food more closely. Usually then comes the great disenchantment where sugar is everywhere and which terms can be used for it.

2. Those who do without sugar will eat the original and unchanged products again. Food is often tested that has never been considered before. Spices are also taking on a completely new role in the preparation of meals. There is an automatic change to a healthier and also to a more natural form of nutrition.

3. After some time without sugar, there is also a positive change in the sense of taste. You notice again that an apple or a banana taste very sweet and individual components of the meal are perceived and tasted more consciously again.

4. Due to the lack of sugar, the blood sugar level also remains in a constant range, which leads to fewer food cravings. It creates a better sense of when you are really hungry and when not.

5. Less sugar also means that you eat healthier foods, experience cravings less often and eat healthier snacks between meals. All of this promotes weight loss.

6. If the blood sugar level drops, this is often expressed as headaches, lack of concentration, nervousness or tremors. These symptoms can be avoided if a sugar-free diet prevents fluctuations in blood sugar levels. Often, not consuming sugar even improves the state of mind and psyche.

Disadvantages of a sugar-free diet

The disadvantages are very minor compared to the advantages, but they have to be mentioned.

1. Since the body gets used to the sugar and it acts like a drug, some withdrawal symptoms occur if you do without it. In the first few days, headaches, tiredness, an increased desire for sweets, mood swings, tremors or even dizziness can occur. But after just a few days, these

negative side effects subside and the positive effects predominate.

2. A sugar-free diet is difficult when you are out and about, when you are invited to dinner or when a meal is due in a restaurant. Usually there are no sugar-free foods or dishes there. Even on vacation, finding sugar-free foods can be very difficult. At home you know over time which products are suitable and which are not. In other grocery stores you first have to find out what can be consumed.

3. Unfortunately, it is very common for people to fail to understand when they mention that they are eating a sugarfree diet. While most people know that eating healthy is important, there is often a lack of understanding. Therefore, one should not be tempted to justify one's diet and negative comments should be ignored.

Sugar-free low-carb recipes
Salads

Balkan salad with cevapcici

<u>Ingredients 4 servings:</u>

- 500 g minced meat, lean
- 170 g onion, red
- 40 g ajvar, mild
- 2 teaspoons of sambal olek
- 1 teaspoon of cumin
- 2 teaspoons of paprika powder, hot pink
- 20 g coconut oil
- salt, pepper
- 4 mini romaine salads
- 300 g paprika, red
- 300 g of cocktail tomatoes
- 300 g avocado
- 300 g of Greek yogurt
- 4 pickles
- 4 tbsp cucumber water
- 4 tbsp ajvar, spicy

<u>Preparation:</u>

1. Cut the pickles into small pieces and mix them with the Greek yoghurt, the

14

cucumber water and the spicy ajvar to
make a dressing. Season it with salt
and pepper.

2. Wash the salads, peppers, and
   tomatoes. Cut the lettuce into small
   pieces. The peppers need to be cut
   into strips. Halve the avocado and
   remove the stone. Cut the pulp into
   pieces. Arrange everything in 4 small
   bowls.

3. Heat the coconut oil in a pan.
   Meanwhile, peel the onion and cut it
   into pieces. Stew the onion and meat
   in the pan. When the meat is crumbly,
   you season it with the mild ajvar, the
   sambal olek, the caraway and the
   paprika powder.

4. Spread the minced meat over the salad
   and pour the dressing over it.

Summer cottage cheese salad

Ingredients 4 servings:

- 600 g of cottage cheese or grainy cream cheese
- 500 g of cocktail tomatoes
- 700 g of cucumber
- 100 g onions, red
- 4 tbsp dill, fresh
- 4 teaspoons of cream horseradish
- 2 tbsp olive oil
- juice of a lime
- 2 teaspoons of birch sugar
- 50 g walnuts
- salt, pepper

Preparation:

1. Wash the small tomatoes and cut them in halves or quarters. Remove the peel from the cucumber and thinly slice it. Skin the onion and finely chop it.
2. Sprinkle the cucumber slices with salt and then place them in a colander. There the slices have to drain for 20-30 minutes. Meanwhile, chop the walnuts into small pieces.
3. Then mix the cottage cheese with the tomatoes, onions, dill, horseradish, oil,

lime juice, birch sugar and nuts. Then fold in the cucumber slices.

4. The salad tastes best when you let it steep overnight.

Pad thai chicken salad

Ingredients 4 servings:

- 800 g chicken fillet
- 1 chilli, red
- 1 clove of garlic
- 1 tbsp sesame oil
- 1/3 red cabbage
- 1/3 pointed cabbage
- 1 onion, red
- 3 carrots
- 1 red pepper
- 1 zucchini
- sea salt, pepper
- pear syrup
- 1 bunch of coriander, fresh
- 150 g yogurt, low in fat
- 50 g peanut cream
- some chili powder
- 100 g coconut

Preparation:

1. Wash the meat well, dry it with a paper towel, and cut it into strips. Rinse, core, and peel the chilli pepper and cut both into small cubes. Mix in the oil

and marinate the meat in it for 30 minutes.

2. Clean the vegetables, then shred the cabbage, onion, and carrots into small pieces. Remove the kernels from the peppers and cut them into sticks along with the zucchini. Mix all the vegetables with salt and pepper and season with the pear syrup. Separate the coriander leaves from the stems. 3. Mix the yogurt with the peanut cream and season the mixture with a little pear syrup, chili powder and salt. Sear the meat in a nonstick pan for 8 minutes until crispy. Arrange the raw vegetables, coriander, and meat on plates and rub the coconut over them. Serve everything with the dressing.

Summer chicken salad

<u>Ingredients 4 servings:</u>

- 100 g currants, black
- 2 chicken breast fillets, approx. 300 g each
- salt, pepper
- 4 onions, red
- 4 tablespoons of olive oil
- 1 head of Lollo Biondo or other leaf salad
- 8 tbsp raspberry vinegar
- 100 g rocket
- 1 bunch of chives

<u>Preparation:</u>

1. Heat the oil in a pan and rinse the meat well. Pat dry and sauté in the hot pan for 5 minutes on each side. Season it with salt and pepper.
2. Skin the onions and cut them into rings. Wash the lettuce well, shake it dry a little, and then tease it. Cut the chives into small rolls and then wash the currants.
3. Take the meat out of the pan and cut it into bite-sized pieces. Then steam the berries briefly in the frying fat and deglaze them with the vinegar. Season everything with salt and pepper.

4. Arrange all the ingredients in small bowls, pour the dressing over them and sprinkle some chives on top.

Ham salad

<u>Ingredients 4 servings:</u>

- 2 hearts of romaine lettuce
- 2 leeks
- 8 tbsp corn, can
- 8 tbsp frozen peas
- 8 slices of cooked ham
- 400 g of yogurt
- 2 tbsp rapeseed oil
- 2 teaspoons of lemon juice
- salt, pepper
- 2 pinches of birch sugar

<u>Preparation:</u>

1. Wash the lettuce and cut it into small pieces. Clean the leek, cut it into thin rings and place it in a salad bowl with the corn and peas.
2. Cut the ham into strips and fold it into the salad.
3. Stir the yogurt, oil, lemon juice and spices into a dressing and spread it over the salad.

Salad boat with an Asian minced meat filling

<u>Ingredients 4 servings:</u>

- 1 ½ cloves of garlic
- ½ chilli
- 1 carrot
- 1 onion, red
- ½ lime
- 1 tbsp rapeseed oil
- 250 g minced meat, pork
- ½ tbsp fish sauce
- ½ tbsp soy sauce, dark without sugar
- 1 tbsp birch sugar
- 1 ½ mini romaine lettuce
- Chili sauce, sugar-free

<u>Preparation:</u>

1. Skin the garlic and finely chop it. Wash the chilli pepper, remove the seeds and cut the half of the pod into small pieces. Peel the carrot and cut it into small cubes. Skin the onion and cut it into rings.
2. Pluck the mint leaves, wash them, and cut some of them into small pieces.
3. Heat the oil in a pan and fry the minced meat in it for 2-3 minutes. Stir

23

in the chilli and garlic and let sear for another minute.

4. Stir in the birch sugar, soy sauce, and fish sauce and continue frying until the minced meat is crispy.

5. Add the carrot, onion, chopped mint leaves and lime juice to the pan and continue frying until the onions are soft. Take the pan off the stove and let everything cool down.

6. Clean the romaine lettuce and remove the leaves. Top the leaves with 1 tablespoon of the ground beef mixture. Cover the meat with the remaining mint leaves and some onion rings. Serve with the chili sauce.

Fruity tomato salad with beef

<u>Ingredients 4 servings:</u>

- 4 beef rump steaks
- 2 tbsp thyme leaves
- 2 tbsp salt flakes
- 1 teaspoon chilli flakes
- 1 teaspoon black pepper
- 650 g tomatoes, ripe
- 2 spring onions
- 2 passion fruits
- 2 stalks of mint
- 8 tbsp olive oil
- 2 tbsp raspberry vinegar
- 1 tbsp balsamic vinegar
- 1 teaspoon maple syrup

<u>Preparation:</u>

1. Rinse the meat under running water and cut it into 1 inch (2.5 cm) strips. Wash and chop the thyme leaves. Crush the salt, chilli flakes, pepper, and thyme leaves with a mortar or chop them on a wooden board.
2. Wash the tomatoes and cut them into small cubes. Wash the spring onions and cut them into rings. Halve the

passion fruit and use a spoon to remove the pulp. Put all of these ingredients in a bowl, then cut the mint into small pieces. 3. For the dressing, mix 4 tablespoons of oil with the balsamic vinegar, raspberry vinegar, maple syrup and 1 teaspoon of the spice mixture. Spread it over the tomato salad.

3. Heat the remaining oil in a pan and fry the strips of meat for 2-3 minutes on each side. Sprinkle the seasoning mixture on top and serve with the tomato salad. Finally, sprinkle the salad with the mint.

Ingredients 4 servings:

- 200 g sliced turkey breast
- 4 spring onions
- 4 peppers, red
- lemon juice
- 1 tbsp Dijon mustard
- 2 tbsp olive oil
- 1 cucumber

Preparation:

1. Wash the peppers, spring onions, and cucumber. Remove the kernels from the peppers. Cut all of the vegetables into cubes.
2. Cut the turkey breast into cubes and mix them with the vegetables in a bowl.
3. Mix the lemon juice with the olive oil and mustard and fold it into the salad. Mix everything together well.
4. Depending on your taste, you can sprinkle the salad with cheese cubes.

Grilled Vegetable Salad

<u>Ingredients 4 servings:</u>

- 200 ml of olive oil
- 3 cloves of garlic
- ½ teaspoon chilli flakes
- 3 heads of romaine lettuce
- 2 heads of radicchio
- 12 cocktail tomatoes
- 6 spring onions
- 12 stalks of asparagus, green
- ½ teaspoon capers
- 2 medium anchovies
- 2 teaspoons of thyme
- 3 tbsp white wine vinegar
- 5 tbsp balsamic vinegar, white
- 1 teaspoon mustard
- 1 medium lemon
- 100 g parmesan cheese
- salt, pepper

<u>Preparation:</u>

1. Pour the olive oil into a bowl and squeeze two peeled garlic cloves into it. Then add the chilli flakes and some salt and pepper. Remove the outer leaves of the lettuce, then cut them in half.

2. Wash the asparagus, tomatoes, and green onions. Then cut them into pieces. Brush the halves of the salads with the remaining oil while heating a grill pan. Put the lettuce in the pan with the oiled side, close it with a lid and fry the lettuce at high temperature for 4 minutes. When it gets brown stripes, add the tomatoes, spring onions and asparagus and sauté these ingredients for 2-3 minutes. You save the rest of the marinade for the dressing.

3. Take the vegetables out of the pan and let them cool. During this time, cut the capers, anchovies and thyme into small pieces and add everything to the bowl that contains the dressing. Press in the third skinned clove of garlic and stir in the vinegar, balsamic vinegar and mustard with a whisk. Season everything with salt and pepper. Add the other ingredients to the bowl, season everything with a large dash of lemon juice and then grate the parmesan over the top.

Spicy leaf salad with mountain cheese

Ingredients 4 servings:

- 6 tbsp white wine vinegar
- salt, pepper
- 1 tbsp honey, liquid
- 1 teaspoon mustard, medium hot
- 4 tbsp oil
- 2 onions, red
- some lettuce leaves of your choice
- 400 g of mountain cheese
- 200 g pickles
- 1 bunch of parsley, fresh

Preparation:

1. For the dressing, mix the honey with the vinegar, salt and pepper. Beat in the oil. Then peel the onions and cut them into narrow wedges. Mix them with the dressing.
2. Wash the lettuce leaves and pluck them into bite-sized pieces. Cut the cheese into strips and the cucumber lengthways into thin slices. Then rinse the parsley under running water and shake it dry. Pluck the leaves and chop

them up. Then mix all the ingredients with the dressing and arrange the salad on plates.

Savory salad with orange and lemon dressing

Ingredients 4 servings:

- 200 g of red lentils
- 600 g savoy cabbage
- 1 orange, organic
- ½ lemon, organic
- 4 tbsp apple cider vinegar
- some sugar
- salt, pepper
- 1 teaspoon oregano, dried
- 4 tablespoons of olive oil
- ½ pomegranate
- 5 stalks of dill
- 1 avocado

Preparation:

1. Bring the lentils to a boil with 600 ml of water and then cook with the lid

closed for 6-8 minutes. Turn down the temperature while doing this. Wash the head of savoy cabbage, cut it into quarters, and remove the stalk. Then cut the leaves into small pieces and place them in a large salad bowl.

2. Rinse the orange and lemon thoroughly with hot water. Rub the peel and squeeze out the juice. Mix the juice with the vinegar, stir in 1 tablespoon of sugar, the dried oregano, and the salt and pepper. Then beat in the oil. Then mix the savoy cabbage with the dressing and the citrus peel. Knead everything well with your hands and let the salad stand for 10-15 minutes.

3. Meanwhile, pour the lentils into a colander and let the water drain off. Cut the pomegranate into quarters, break them into pieces and remove the seeds. Wash the dill, shake it dry, and chop it up.

4. Divide the avocado in half, remove the stone, and use a spoon to remove the pulp before cutting it into small cubes. Then mix the lentils with the seeds of the pomegranate, dill, avocado and savoy cabbage.

Soups

Vegetable soup from Greece

<u>Ingredients 4 servings:</u>

- 1 medium onion
- 1 clove of garlic
- 1 stick of celery
- 1 medium carrot
- ½ tbsp olive oil
- 250 ml of vegetable stock
- 500 ml of water
- 300 g canned tomatoes
- 100 g lentils, dry
- 1/3 teaspoon thyme
- 1/3 teaspoon basil

<u>Preparation:</u>

1. Remove the peel from the onion and the clove of garlic and chop them up. Wash the celery, peel the carrot and cut everything into small cubes.
2. Heat the olive oil in a medium saucepan and sauté the onion cubes for 2-3 minutes. Then fry the carrot, garlic and celery for 3-4 minutes as well.

3. Pour the vegetable stock and water into the pot. Add the remaining ingredients and bring the soup to a boil. Then reduce the temperature and let the vegetable soup simmer gently for 15-20 minutes. Once the lentils are soft, you can serve the soup.

Creamy and light asparagus soup

<u>Ingredients 4 servings:</u>

- 3 tbsp almond flakes
- 500 ml of milk
- 250 ml of vegetable stock
- 750 g asparagus, green
- 1 bunch of spring onions
- 1 pinch of cayenne pepper
- 1 teaspoon tarragon
- 4 tbsp crème fraîche

<u>Preparation:</u>

1. Toast the almond flakes in a non-stick pan for 5 minutes. Make sure that they don't burn and therefore choose a low temperature level.
2. Heat the milk and broth in a saucepan. Meanwhile, peel the asparagus and wash the spring onions. Cut both into pieces and let them cook for 20 minutes in the vegetable stock and milk mixture.
3. Then take the pot off the stove, puree the soup with a hand blender and season with the cayenne pepper and tarragon.

4. Before serving, stir in the crème fraîche and sprinkle the soup with the toasted almonds.

Sharp bean pot

<u>Ingredients 4 servings:</u>

- 100 g onion, red
- 500 g green beans
- 500 g paprika, colored
- 400 g of chunky tomatoes
- 300 ml of vegetable stock
- 1 can of kidney beans
- 2 teaspoons of paprika powder, noble sweet
- 2 teaspoons of paprika powder, hot pink
- 1 tbsp marjoram, dried
- 2 teaspoons of sambal olek
- 2 teaspoons of birch sugar
- 150 g of cream cheese
- 15 ml of olive oil
- salt, pepper

<u>Preparation:</u>

1. Remove the skin from the onions and chop them up. Heat the olive oil in a saucepan and sweat the diced onion in it. Wash the peppers and cut them into cubes. Fry the diced pepper and the beans in the pan for 2-3 minutes. Pour in the broth and the chunky tomatoes.

2. Stir in the spices and the sambal olek as well as the birch sugar and let everything simmer gently for 10 minutes. Then drain the kidney beans and add them to the pot. Stir in the cream cheese and season the bean pot with salt and pepper.

Cream of Leek Soup

underline>Ingredients 4 servings:</u>

- 15 g coconut oil
- 1-2 onions
- 1 clove of garlic
- 150 g of carrots
- 150 g parsnips
- 500 g leeks
- 900 ml of vegetable stock
- 175 ml of cream
- 3-4 teaspoons of cream horseradish
- 250 g of crabs
- salt, pepper

Preparation:

1. Skin the onion and garlic and dice them both. Heat the oil in a saucepan and steam the onion cubes in it until translucent. Add the garlic and cook for 1 minute.
2. Peel the carrots and parsnips and wash the leeks. Cut the root vegetables into cubes and the leek into rings. Then put the vegetables in the pot and sweat them briefly. Pour the broth on it and let the soup simmer for 20 minutes. Then puree them with a hand blender and stir in both the cream and the horseradish.

3. Then stir the crabs into the soup, season them with salt and pepper and heat them up again for 5 minutes.

4. If the soup is too thick, you can add a little more broth.

Pizza and Vegetable Soup

<u>Ingredients 4 servings:</u>

- 20 ml of olive oil
- 100 g onions, red
- 700 g zucchini
- 300 peppers, red or orange
- 300 g mushrooms
- 500 g of cocktail tomatoes
- 2 teaspoons oregano, dried
- 160 g pepperoni salami
- 4 teaspoons of tomato pesto
- 200 g mozzarella
- 50 g parmesan cheese, grated

<u>Preparation:</u>

1. Skin the onion, wash the peppers, zucchini, and cherry tomatoes. Clean the mushrooms. Cut the pepper, onion, and salami into cubes. Grate the zucchini with a kitchen grater. Cut the tomatoes into quarters and the mushrooms into slices.
2. Heat the oil in a saucepan and sweat the onion cubes in it until translucent. Add the salami, shredded zucchini, bell pepper and mushrooms and sauté everything for 2-3 minutes. Fold in the tomatoes and oregano

and let the soup simmer for another 5-6 minutes. Keep stirring while doing this.

3. Then add the pesto. Drain the mozzarella and cut it into cubes. Then add it to the soup along with the parmesan. Let the cheese melt for only 2-3 minutes.

4. Season the soup with salt and pepper and serve.

Tomato soup with salmon

<u>Ingredients 4 servings:</u>

- 15 ml of olive oil
- 75 g onions
- 150 g celery
- 750 ml of tomato puree
- 400 g of peeled tomatoes
- 500 ml of vegetable stock
- 100 g frozen mango, without sugar
- 300 g frozen salmon
- 70 g of cream cheese
- 1 teaspoon balsamic vinegar, light
- salt, pepper

<u>Preparation:</u>

1. Heat the olive oil in a large stock pot. Skin the onion, cut it into small cubes and sauté it in the hot oil until translucent. Wash the celery, dice it and add it to the onion. Sweat him up.
2. Extinguish everything with the passed tomatoes and the peeled tomatoes and pour in the vegetable stock. Add the frozen mango pieces and let the soup simmer for 20 minutes. Then puree them with a hand blender.

3. Put the defrosted salmon with the balsamic vinegar and cream cheese in a blender and puree it to a smooth mass. Season them with salt and pepper and then add them to the soup in portions. Use a teaspoon for the correct size. Let the small dumplings soak in the soup for 7-8 minutes without it boiling. Then season again with salt and pepper.

Vegetable soup with chicken

Ingredients 3-4 servings:

- 900 ml of vegetable stock
- 1 leg of chicken
- 1 chicken breast fillet
- 15 g coconut oil
- 1 onion, red
- 1 clove of garlic
- ½ tsp curry paste
- 250 g parsnips
- 250 g leeks
- 2 carrots
- 150 ml coconut milk
- 100 ml orange juice, fresh
- 2 teaspoons of curry powder
- ¼ teaspoon cinnamon, ground
- salt, pepper

Preparation:

1. Heat the vegetable stock in a saucepan and cook the chicken leg and chicken breast in it for 20-25 minutes. Then take the meat out again, remove the meat from the leg and cut everything into small pieces.
2. Skin the onion and clove of garlic and cut them into small cubes. Heat the

45

coconut oil in a large saucepan and steam the onion in it until translucent. Add the garlic and curry paste and fry both briefly.

3. Peel the parsnip, leek, and carrot and cut the carrot and parsnip into cubes. Cut the leek into rings and fry everything for 2-3 minutes.

4. Then remove the vegetables from the meat with the broth and let them simmer for 15 minutes. Then puree the soup with a hand blender and stir in the coconut milk and freshly squeezed orange juice.

5. Finally, season the soup with the curry powder and cinnamon as well as with salt and pepper. Stir in the chicken and reheat the soup just before serving.

Asian soup with chicken

<u>Ingredients 4 servings:</u>

- 1 zucchini, green
- 1 zucchini, yellow
- 2 carrots
- 3 spring onions
- 1 clove of garlic
- 1 piece of ginger
- 400 g of chicken breast fillet
- 4 tablespoons of olive oil
- 3 teaspoons of chicken broth
- salt, pepper
- 1.2 liters of water
- ½ bunch of coriander
- ½ bunch of Thai basil
- 2 limes, organic

<u>Preparation:</u>

1. Wash the zucchini and use the spiral cutter to cut into thin noodles. Peel the carrots and make pasta too. Rinse the spring onions well and cut the white part into cubes. You cut the green of the onion into rings. Skin the garlic, peel the ginger and chop it very finely.

47

2. Wash the meat well, pat it dry with kitchen paper, and cut it into slices. Heat 2 tablespoons of oil in a saucepan and fry the spring onions, ginger and garlic in it for 1-2 minutes. Pour in the water and stir in the broth. Now put the meat in the pot and let the soup simmer gently for 12-15 minutes. Add the vegetable noodles 5 minutes before the end of the cooking time.
3. Wash the herbs, shake them dry, and chop half of the coriander leaves. Pluck half of the basil leaves and cut them very small as well.
4. Rinse the limes well under hot water and cut them in half. Squeeze out the juice of 1 lime, cut the other into wedges.
5. Wash the chili peppers, remove the seeds, and chop them into large pieces. Put the lime juice, chopped herbs and 2 tablespoons of oil in a blender and puree everything into a paste
6. Season the soup with salt and pepper and serve with the chili paste.

Meat dishes

Low carb ham pizza

<u>Ingredients 1 pizza:</u>

- 1 ½ cans of tuna
- 3 eggs
- 100 g mushrooms
- 3 slices of cooked ham
- 80 g cheese, grated
- 200 ml of tomato puree
- Italian herbs
- salt, pepper
- oregano

<u>Preparation:</u>

1. Beat two eggs in a bowl and stir well. Drain the juice from the tuna well and mix it with the eggs. Spread the mixture in a circle on a baking sheet lined with baking paper until a 4-6 mm thick base is formed.
2. Bake the base in the oven for 10-15 minutes at a temperature of 180 ° C top / bottom heat.
3. Mix the tomatoes with the Italian herbs and season the sauce with salt and pepper.

4. Take the bottom out of the oven and brush it with the tomato sauce. Cut the ham into pieces and spread it on the pizza.

5. Roughly sour the mushrooms, cut them into slices and spread them on the pizza as well. Sprinkle the cheese on top.

6. Beat the last egg and put it on the pizza.

7. Place the baking sheet in the oven for 20 minutes, until the cheese has melted and the egg has hardened.

8. Sprinkle the pizza with some pizza seasoning before serving.

Grilled pork loin with zucchini vegetables

Ingredients 4 servings:

- 1 kg of pork loin
- 140 g of bacon
- 900 g zucchini
- 2 tbsp olive oil
- ½ chilli pepper
- 2 teaspoons of rosemary
- 2 teaspoons of thyme
- 4 cloves of garlic
- 1 teaspoon pepper
- ½ teaspoon salt
- some toothpicks

Preparation:

1. Cut the loin into thicker slices. Place the bacon side by side on a plate.
2. Skin the garlic and press it into a bowl. Stir in the olive oil and season the marinade with the spices.
3. Place the loin slices on top of the bacon and brush them with the marinade. Then wrap the bacon around the meat and secure it with a toothpick.

4. Place the loins on the grill or in a grill pan and grill them all around. When they're crispy, you can take them off the grill and wrap them in aluminum foil. Now place the meat packets on the edge of the grill and let them rest for 15 minutes.
5. In the meantime, wash the zucchini and cut them into thin strips with a peeler. Put these on the grill and season them with a little salt and pepper.
6. Place the zucchini strips on a plate, serve the loin next to them.

Tender fillet of beef with a side of chicory

<u>Ingredients 4 servings:</u>

- 30 g pumpkin seeds   - 1 tbsp sesame seeds
- 500 g beef tenderloin
- 6 tbsp olive oil
- sea salt, pepper
- 2 tbsp sunflower oil
- 200 g of cocktail tomatoes
- 4 stalks of thyme
- 1 tbsp balsamic vinegar, dark
- 2 tbsp red wine vinegar
- 2 tbsp pumpkin seed oil
- 600 g chicory
- 20 g butter
- 1 tbsp lemon juice
- 1 tbsp chives rolls

<u>Preparation:</u>

1. Preheat the oven to 160 ° C fan-assisted.
2. Chop the pumpkin seeds and mix them with the sesame seeds in a small bowl. Rub the meat with ½ tablespoon of olive oil and then season with pepper. Turn the fillets in the pumpkin and sesame mixture.
3. Heat the sunflower oil in a pan and fry the meat on both sides over medium heat.

53

Then take it out of the pan and place it on a baking sheet. The meat must now cook in the middle of the oven for 25-30 minutes.

4. After ¼ hour mix the washed tomatoes with 1 tablespoon of olive oil and the thyme and spread them on the baking sheet as well.

5. Mix the balsamic vinegar with the red wine vinegar, 4 tablespoons of olive oil, the pumpkin seed oil, sea salt and the pepper.

6. Remove the end leaves from the chicory and cut it into quarters. **Do not** cut out the stalk.

7. Heat the butter and 1 tablespoon of olive oil in a pan and add the salad. Fry the chicory until it turns light brown. Then season it with salt, pepper and a little lemon juice.

8. Take the meat and cherry tomatoes out of the oven and let them cool for 5 minutes. Meanwhile, place the chicory in the oven to keep it warm.

9. Cut the beef fillet into slices and serve it on plates with the tomatoes and chicory. Drizzle some dressing over it and sprinkle the dish with the chives.

Goulash with Kasseler

<u>Ingredients 4 servings:</u>

- 2 peppers, red
- 1 bell pepper, yellow
- 3 onions
- 4 cloves of garlic
- 600 g pork loin, boneless
- some star anise, ground
- 3 tablespoons of olive oil
- salt, pepper
- 1 tbsp tomato paste
- 1 tbsp paprika powder, noble sweet
- 1 tbsp paprika powder, hot
- 400 ml of vegetable stock
- 1 tbsp sauce thickener, light

<u>Preparation:</u>

1. Wash all the peppers, remove the seeds, cut them into quarters and then into narrow strips. Remove the peel from the onions, cut them in half and cut them into strips. Skin the garlic and cut it into thin slices. Rinse the meat well under running water and cut it into bite-sized pieces.

2. Heat the oil in a roasting pan and fry the pepper strips, onions and garlic in it. Season the whole thing with a little star anise, salt and pepper.
3. Stir in the tomato paste and the sweet and hot paprika powder. Roast these ingredients briefly. Fill up with the broth and now add the meat. Then let everything cook for 1012 minutes at medium temperature.
4. Stir in the sauce thickener and briefly boil the goulash. As soon as the desired consistency is reached, you can serve the Kasseler Goulash.

Ingredients 4 servings:

- 2 onions
- 200 g mushrooms
- 2 cans of artichokes
- 4 thyme stalks
- 6 tbsp olive oil
- 4 chicken breast fillets
- 200 ml of chicken broth
- salt, pepper
- 4 stalks of parsley
- 40 g parmesan cheese

Preparation:

1. Skin the onions and cut them into rings. Carefully clean the mushrooms and cut them in half. Pour the artichokes into a colander, drain the liquid well, and cut it in half. Pluck the thyme leaves and wash them.
2. Heat 2 tablespoons of oil in a pan and sear the meat on
3. both sides. Then take it out of the pan and steam the onions in the frying fat for 5 minutes until they are soft.
4. Now pour the remaining olive oil into the pan and sear the mushrooms.

Deglaze them with the broth, then add the artichokes, thyme and chicken. Season everything with salt and pepper and let it simmer gently for ¼ hour.

5. Separate the leaves from the stems of the parsley and chop them up. If you don't have grated parmesan, finely slice it. Then sprinkle the vegetables with the meat and the mushrooms with the parsley and parmesan and serve the dish.

Parmesan pork schnitzel

<u>Ingredients 4 servings:</u>

- 2 eggs
- 40 g parmesan cheese, grated
- 10 tbsp oil
- 4 pork schnitzel, thin
- 6 tbsp vinegar
- salt, pepper
- 6 tbsp vinegar
- 1 kg of tomatoes
- 4 tbsp parsley, chopped

<u>Preparation:</u>

1. Whisk the 2 eggs with the parmesan and season the schnitzel with salt and pepper. Heat 5 tablespoons of oil in a pan.
2. Meanwhile, transfer the egg mixture to a flat plate and toss the schnitzel in it. Then put the meat directly in the hot pan and fry them on both sides for 5 minutes at a medium temperature until they have a golden brown crust.
3. Mix the vinegar with the remaining olive oil and season the mixture with salt and pepper. Wash the tomatoes, remove the roots of the tomatoes, and

cut them into wedges. Mix them with the chopped parsley into the oil and vinegar mixture.

4. Take the schnitzel out of the pan and place them on kitchen paper. Sprinkle them with a little parmesan and serve with the tomato salad.

Fried beef skewers

<u>Ingredients 4 servings:</u>

- 4 beef rump steaks (approx. 600 g)
- 10 tbsp soy sauce
- 2 tbsp lime juice
- 1 teaspoon chilli flakes
- 500 g of carrots
- 1 Chinese cabbage
- 6 tbsp oil
- 4 tbsp peanuts, roasted and salted
- 12 stalks of coriander
- wooden skewers

1. <u>Preparation:</u>

    1. Cut the beef into oblong strips and place them on the wooden skewers as a wave. Then stir together the soy sauce, the juice of the lime and the chilli flakes.
    2. Place the meat skewers in a dish, spread the sauce mixture over it and let them marinate for ½ hour.
    3. Meanwhile, peel the carrots and cut them into 4 cm thin strips. Wash the Chinese cabbage, cut it into quarters and remove the stalk. Then cut the quarters into strips.
    4. Take the meat out of the marinade and pat it dry. Heat 4 tablespoons of oil in a pan and fry the

skewers for 2 minutes over medium heat. Then take them out of the pan and keep them warm.

5. Now add the carrot sticks and 2 more tablespoons of oil to the pan and sear them while stirring for 2 minutes. Add the Chinese cabbage and let the vegetables sear again for 1 minute.

6. Mix the marinade of the meat with 10 tablespoons of water and use it to deglaze the vegetables in the pan. Let the liquid boil once. Place the skewers on the vegetables and heat them up briefly.

7. Then chop the nuts and coriander into large pieces. Arrange the beef skewers with the Chinese cabbage on plates and sprinkle them with some peanuts and the coriander.

Pork medallions with cauliflower

Ingredients 4 servings:

- 1 kg of cauliflower
- 300 g of cocktail tomatoes
- 600 g pork tenderloin
- 160 g butter
- 2 egg yolks
- 4 tbsp cream yogurt
- 15 basil leaves
- 4 tbsp oil
- salt, cayenne pepper

Preparation:

1. Wash the cauliflower, divide it, and blanch it in boiling salted water for 6 minutes. Then drain the water and let the cauliflower drain.
2. Wash the tomatoes and meat under running water. Cut the fillet into 2 cm wide slices.
3. Put the butter in a saucepan and let it melt. Briefly boil them. Separate the eggs and put the egg yolks, cream yoghurt and basil leaves in a tall container and puree everything with a hand blender. Stir in the hot butter while you continue to mash with the

hand blender. Then season the mixture with salt and pepper.

4. Heat the oil in a non-stick pan and fry the meat for 2-3 minutes on both sides until it has turned a light brown color. Take it out of the pan.

5. Then put the tomatoes and cauliflower in the pan, fry both for about 5 minutes and season with a little salt.

6. Arrange the meat with the cauliflower on plates and pour the sauce over them.

Cheese meat rolls

Ingredients 4 servings:

- 1 kg of minced meat, mixed
- ½ pack of sliced cheese, butter cheese
- 2 packets of bacon
- 500 ml of pureed tomatoes
- 1 onion
- 1 clove of garlic
- salt, pepper
- 4 tbsp crème fraîche

Preparation:

1. Lay the cheese slices on top of each other and cut them into strips.
2. Take a handful of the meat off at a time, press it flat and place a strip of cheese in the middle. Roll up the ground beef until the cheese is well enclosed in the ground beef. Then wrap 2 strips of bacon around each roll.
3. Place the rolls in a pan and fry them well all around.
4. Meanwhile, peel the onion and garlic, cut both into small pieces and sweat them in the frying fat. Pour in the tomatoes and

stir in the crème fraîche. Season the sauce with salt and pepper.

5. Take the meat rolls out of the pan and serve them with the sauce.

Savoy cabbage mince rolls with cauliflower puree

Ingredients 4 servings:

- 1 savoy cabbage
- 400 g of minced meat
- salt, pepper
- Nutmeg, ground
- 3 tbsp crème fraîche
- 150 ml of vegetable stock
- 1 cauliflower
- 250 ml of milk
- ½ tbsp vegetable stock, powder
- 1 tbsp chia seeds
- 1 tbsp almond flour

Preparation:

1. Divide the cauliflower into florets and cook it in salted boiling water until it is firm to the bite.
2. Separate the outer large savoy cabbage leaves. Use a sharp knife to cut the hard and thick part of the stalk flat.
3. Take the smaller savoy cabbage leaves and chop them very finely. Briefly blanch the large leaves in salted boiling water so that the leaves can be rolled up better.

67

4. Mix the minced meat with the crème fraîche, the chopped savoy cabbage and the spices. Then cover the large leaves with the minced meat mixture and roll them up. Then put them in a pan.

5. Pour the vegetable stock over the rolls and steam them for 35 minutes with the lid closed.

6. Drain the cauliflower. Briefly boil the milk with the vegetable stock powder, some grated nutmeg, the chia seeds and the almond flour. Puree the cauliflower with a hand blender and mix it with the sauce.

7. Arrange the minced meat rolls on a plate and serve with the cauliflower puree.

Stuffed chicken breast fillet with bacon

<u>Ingredients 4 servings:</u>

- 1 kg of chicken breast fillet
- 200 g bacon strips
- 160 g of feta cheese
- 4 sun-dried tomatoes
- 20 olives, black without a core
- 2 sprigs of rosemary
- 2 cloves of garlic
- 4 teaspoons of olive oil

<u>Preparation:</u>

1. Wash the rosemary and peel the garlic cloves. Then cut the sun-dried tomatoes, rosemary, cloves of garlic, olives and cheese into small pieces and stir everything in a bowl with the olive oil.
2. Use a sharp knife to cut the chicken breast fillets on the side to make a pocket. Fill the bag with the filling and seal it. If the opening doesn't stay closed properly, you can fix it with a toothpick.
3. Wrap the stuffed pieces of meat in the bacon. Then the chicken breast fillets are fried in a grill pan or on the grill.
4. A crunchy salad is ideal as a side dish.

Indian curry with chicken

<u>Ingredients 4 servings:</u>

- 1 onion
- 1 clove of garlic
- 3 tomatoes
- 500 g chicken breast fillet
- 2 tbsp olive oil
- 1-2 tbsp curry powder
- 1 can of coconut milk
- 250 g spinach
- salt, pepper

1. <u>Preparation:</u>

   1. Peel the onion and clove of garlic and cut them into small cubes. Then press the garlic with a press. Rinse the tomatoes well and dice them. Also, after washing the meat, cut the meat into larger cubes.
   2. Take a pan, pour in the olive oil, heat it and fry the meat in it for 4-5 minutes. Always turn it with a spatula. After about 2 minutes, sprinkle the curry powder over it and sauté the meat again briefly. Add the diced tomatoes to the frying pan, let all the ingredients cook together for 3-4 minutes before adding the coconut milk. Let the curry simmer gently for 10 minutes.

3. Wash the spinach leaves, shake them dry, and add them to the pan. Wait for him to collapse. Season the curry pot with salt and pepper.

Low carb burger

Ingredients 4 servings:

Gold flaxseed bun:

- 100 g almonds, ground
- 50 g (gold) flaxseed flour
- 30 g butter
- 3 eggs
- 5 g psyllium husk powder
- 100 g of Greek yogurt
- 1 teaspoon baking powder
- 1 pinch of salt

Burger:

- 4 slices of butter cheese
- 2-3 tomatoes
- 4 leaves of iceberg lettuce
- 800 g minced meat, beef
- salt, pepper
- 80 g mayonnaise

Preparation:

1. Preheat your oven to 175 ° C with a fan oven.
2. Put all the ingredients for the bun dough in a large bowl and mix them with a mixer

or food processor to form a smooth dough.

3. Cover a baking sheet with parchment paper and then form 4 rolls out of the dough. Place them on the baking sheet and bake them in the oven for ½ hour.

4. Take the buns out of the oven and let them cool.

5. Then season the minced meat with salt and pepper and shape it into meat coins that are about 1 cm thick.

6. Cut the buns open and brush the mayonnaise on both sides. Wash the lettuce leaves and tomatoes. Cut the tomatoes into 8 slices.

7. First cover the lower half of the roll with the lettuce leaf and spread 2 tomato slices on top. Repeat this process for all buns.

8. Heat some oil in a pan and fry the meat coins in it for 2 minutes on both sides. Then place a slice of cheese on each meat in the pan so that it melts easily.

9. Then take the meat out of the pan and cover the bun halves with it. Close the burgers with the top half and serve.

Ingredients 4 servings:

- 1 kg of zucchini
- 200 g celery
- 100 g of carrots
- 25 g butter
- ½ onion
- 400 g chopped tomatoes, can
- 250 ml red wine, dry
- 1 kg of minced meat
- 50 ml of olive oil
- ½ clove of garlic
- 100 g of bacon
- 50 g parmesan cheese
- salt, pepper
- 1-2 sprigs of rosemary
- 1-2 sprigs of thyme
- 1 tbsp birch sugar

Preparation:

1. Heat the butter and oil in a saucepan. Meanwhile, remove the skin from the onion. Chop the bacon and onions and fry them in the saucepan.
2. Peel the celery and carrots, cut everything into small pieces and add it to the pot as

well. Skin the garlic and press it into the pot.

3. Then fry the minced meat in the pot. Chop the rosemary and thyme sprigs and add them to the meat. Rub everything off with the red wine.

4. Pour in the tomatoes and stir in the birch sugar. Let the Bolognese simmer for 2 hours at a low temperature.

5. Then season the sauce with salt and pepper.

6. Meanwhile, wash the zucchini and use a spiral cutter to cut them into noodles. Then add them to the sauce for 15 minutes.

7. Grate the parmesan and sprinkle with the zucchini noodles and Bolognese before serving.

Indian curry chicken

<u>Ingredients 4 servings:</u>

- 600 g chicken breast fillet
- ½ onion
- 2 cloves of garlic
- 1 teaspoon tomato paste
- 50 g butter
- 1 tbsp curry powder
- 2 teaspoons of cumin
- 2 teaspoons of coriander, ground
- 2 teaspoons of paprika powder, noble sweet
- 1 teaspoon turmeric
- ½ teaspoon cinnamon
- ¼ teaspoon ginger, ground
- ½ teaspoon pepper
- 400 ml of coconut milk
- 800 g of cauliflower

<u>Preparation:</u>

1. Rinse the meat under running water and cut it into pieces. Remove the skin from the onion and garlic cloves and chop them both into small pieces. Then mix the onion and garlic cubes in a bowl with all the spices.

2. Melt the butter in a saucepan and sweat the onion and garlic mixture in it for 3 minutes. Then add the chicken and coconut milk and let everything simmer for 30 minutes. Then taste with salt.

3. Meanwhile, remove the stalk from the cauliflower and finely grate it with a food processor or grater. Then briefly toast the cauliflower rice in a little water or a little oil in the pan.

4. Serve the wrong rice with the curry.

Mushroom Chili Pot

<u>Ingredients 4 servings:</u>

- 2 boxes of mushrooms
- 2 onions
- 2 cloves of garlic
- 400 g ground beef
- 4 tbsp tomato paste
- 2 cans of tomatoes, chopped
- 2 chili peppers
- 400 ml of vegetable stock
- 1 pack of sour cream
- salt, pepper
- paprika powder

<u>Preparation:</u>

1. Peel the onions and garlic and core the chili peppers. Chop everything up and sauté it in a pan with a little hot oil. 2. Meanwhile, clean the mushrooms and cut them into slices.
2. As soon as the onions are translucent, add the minced meat and fry it until it's done. Then add the mushrooms and continue to fry everything until

the mushrooms turn brown. 4. Mix the vegetable stock and pour it into the pan, along with the chopped tomatoes and tomato paste. Season the chilli with salt, pepper, and paprika powder.

3. Take the pan off the heat, let the chilli cool down a bit and finally stir in the sour cream.

Chorizo scrambled eggs

Ingredients 4 servings:

- 1 red pepper
- 2 spring onions
- 150 g of chorizo
- 1 tbsp olive oil
- 6 eggs
- 4 tbsp milk
- salt, pepper

Preparation:

1. Wash the pepper, remove the seeds, and cut them into small cubes. Clean the spring onions and cut them into rings. Then halve the chorizo lengthways and cut it into slices. Heat the olive oil in a pan and fry the sausage in it for 6 minutes. Keep turning them over and over.
2. After 3 minutes, add the diced paprika and spring onions. 3. Meanwhile, whisk the milk and eggs together and season the mixture with salt and pepper. Add the mixture to the pan and let it set. You have to stir carefully

with a spatula over and over again.
Serve the scrambled eggs.

Tomato eggs out of the oven

Ingredients 4 servings:

- 1 medium onion
- 2 cloves of garlic
- 1 medium bell pepper, yellow
- 1 medium bell pepper, red
- 1 tsp harissa spice paste
- ½ teaspoon paprika powder, noble sweet
- 400 g of chunky tomatoes, can
- 1 handful of parsley, fresh
- 1 teaspoon salt
- 4 medium eggs

Preparation:

1. Remove the skin from the onions and garlic cloves and chop them into small pieces. Wash the peppers and cut them into strips. Then preheat the oven to 180 ° C fan-assisted air. 2. Take a pan and add the onions, garlic, harissa seasoning, paprika strips, and paprika powder. Bring all of the ingredients to a boil until the pepper strips are tender. Scatter the chopped parsley and season with salt.

2. Use a spoon to make small hollows in the vegetables and slide one egg into each. Then place the pan in the oven for 4 minutes until the egg white has set.
3. Garnish the egg pan with a little parsley before serving.

Fake asparagus risotto with cauliflower

<u>Ingredients 4 servings:</u>

- 1 kg of cauliflower
- 100 g of onions
- 400 g asparagus, green
- 150 g avocado, ripe
- 50 g rocket, organic
- 130 g goat cheese with fenugreek
- 120 g goat cream cheese
- salt, pepper
- 15 ml of olive oil

<u>Preparation:</u>

1. Wash the cauliflower and roughly grate it. Heat the olive oil in a saucepan while cutting the peeled onion into small cubes. Steam them translucent in the hot oil.
2. Peel the asparagus and cut it into bite-sized pieces. Add the cauliflower and asparagus to the saucepan, season with salt and pepper and cook for 8-10 minutes.
3. Stir in the goat cheese and fresh goat cheese and wait for both to melt.
4. Halve the avocado, remove the stone and cut the pulp into small pieces. Then add them to the saucepan and mix everything

together well. Season to taste with salt and pepper and then turn off the stove.

5. Wash the rocket, shake it dry and fold it into the risotto.

Fried kohlrabi with spinach cheese paste

Ingredients 4 servings:

- 1.5 kg of kohlrabi
- 500 g young spinach, frozen
- 250 grams of gorgonzola
- 200 g of cream cheese
- 20 g coconut oil
- salt, pepper

Preparation:

1. Peel the kohlrabi and cut it into large cubes. Heat a little coconut oil and fry the kohlrabi in it. Keep stirring it until it has turned a little brown.
2. Heat the remaining coconut oil in another saucepan and let the spinach thaw in it. Add the cream cheese so that it can dissolve in the warmth of the spinach. Stir in the gorgonzola until it's melted too. Season everything with salt and pepper and serve the fried kohlrabi with the spinach and cheese cream.

Refreshing gazpacho

<u>Ingredients 4 servings:</u>

- 1 kg of tomatoes, fresh or canned
- 2 medium cucumbers
- 4 tablespoons of olive oil
- 4 tbsp vinegar
- 2 cloves of garlic
- 4 ice cubes
- salt, pepper

<u>Preparation:</u>

1. Wash the tomatoes and cucumbers and cut them into cubes. Pour the oil and vinegar into a blender and add the peeled garlic and ice cubes. Puree everything to a smooth mass and season with salt and pepper. Alternatively, you can puree the ingredients with a hand blender.
2. If you want, you can put some chopped tomato and cucumber cubes as a topping on the gazpacho.

Ingredients 4 servings:

- 2 medium lemons
- 4 tablespoons of olive oil
- 500 g halloumi
- 8 teaspoons of olive tapenade
- 8 teaspoons of grilled peppers, pickled

Preparation:

1. Cut the lemons in half and rub off the peel from two halves. Then squeeze out the two halves. Cut the other two halves into 8 slices.
2. Mix the lemon zest with the juice and oil. Place the lemon slices with the cheese in a bowl and spread the marinade over them. The cheese then has to steep for 30 minutes.
3. Then place the cheese with the lemon slices on a grill or put it in a grill pan and roast it on both sides for 2 minutes. 4. Arrange the cheese on plates and sprinkle it with the tapenade, the dressing and top it with the pickled peppers.

Broccoli Cheese Omelette

Ingredients 4 servings:

- 1.2 kg broccoli, fresh
- 12 medium eggs
- 4 drops of milk
- 1 clove of garlic
- 2 medium shallots
- 240 g cheese, grated
- salt, pepper
- some olive oil

Preparation:

1. Bring a saucepan of salted water to a boil and cook the broccoli in it until it is firm to the bite. Skin and chop the garlic and shallots. In a tall container, stir the eggs and milk together with a whisk.
2. Pour a little olive oil into a pan, heat it up, and add the garlic, broccoli, and shallots. Briefly toss the vegetables in the pan and then pour in the egg-milk mixture. Let the eggs set on medium heat for a few minutes.
3. Sprinkle the grated cheese over the omelette, season it with salt and pepper, and then slide it out of the pan

onto a plate. Depending on your taste, you can fold the omelette on top of each other in the middle.

Mexican vegetable frittata

<u>Ingredients 4 servings:</u>

- 8 medium eggs
- 75 ml of milk
- 100 g chili peppers, pickled
- 3 spring onions
- 100 g Edam
- salt, pepper

<u>Preparation:</u>

1. Preheat the oven to 190 ° C and brush a baking dish with a little oil.
2. Whisk the eggs with the milk and cut the chili peppers into small pieces. Wash the spring onions, chop them up and grate the cheese. Put all the ingredients in the baking dish, pour the egg-milk mixture over it and season with salt and pepper.
3. Place the pan in the oven for 25 minutes, until the egg has set. Then divide the frittata into 4 servings and serve.

Fried chard and tomato pan with egg

<u>Ingredients 4 servings:</u>

- 500 g of cocktail tomatoes
- 2 tbsp red wine vinegar
- 2 kg of Swiss chard
- 4 medium onions
- 8 cloves of garlic
- 4 tablespoons of olive oil
- 8 medium eggs
- salt, pepper

<u>Preparation:</u>

1. Wash the small tomatoes, cut them all in half once, then quarter them and place them in a salad bowl with the red wine vinegar. Mix the two ingredients together and set the bowl aside for now.
2. Cut the stalks from the chard, set them aside, and wash the leaves well. Then place them in a colander so that the excess water can drain off. As soon as they have dried a little, you have to roughly chop the leaves. Then cut the stems into thin strips. Skin the onions and garlic and cut everything into small cubes.

3. Heat the oil in a pan. Add the onions and the finely chopped stems and sauté them for 10 minutes. Turn down the temperature a little, add the garlic and sauté everything for 1 minute. Stir well while doing this. Then put the leaves of the chard in the pan and season everything with salt and pepper. Now turn the temperature to the highest level and wait until the leaves have collapsed. Stir vigorously as you do this.

4. Then lower the temperature a little and use a spoon to make 4 indentations in the vegetables. There you have to slide 1 egg into each. Then put a lid on the pan and let the eggs set for 4 minutes.

5. At the end, spread the red wine vinegar tomatoes on top and serve the dish.

Ingredients 4 servings:

- 8 giant mushrooms
- 1 shallot
- 2 cloves of garlic
- 2 tbsp oil
- 60 g pine nuts
- 1 bunch of rocket
- 120 g blue cheese
- salt, pepper

Preparation:

1. Preheat the oven to 200 ° C top and bottom heat.
2. Roughly clean the mushrooms, unscrew the stems and carefully hollow out the heads. Skin the shallot and the garlic cloves and chop them up. Then cut the stems very small too.
   3. Put the oil in a pan, heat it and fry the shallot, garlic, mushroom stalks and pine nuts until golden brown.
3. Rinse the arugula, shake it dry, and chop it up. Mix the fried ingredients from the pan and the chopped cheese into the rocket. Then season everything with salt and pepper.

95

4. Pour the mixture into the mushrooms, spread them on a baking sheet and let them gratin in the oven for 20-25 minutes.

Onioncake

<u>Ingredients 1 cake:</u>

- 500 g onions
- 50 g butter
- 200 g cheese, grated
- 150 g bacon cubes or ham cubes
- 100 g almond flour
- 5 eggs
- 150 ml of milk
- Ground caraway seeds
- salt, pepper

<u>Preparation:</u>

1. Preheat your oven to 200 ° C top / bottom heat and coat a springform pan with a little butter.
2. Remove the skin from the onion and cut it into thin rings. Heat the butter in a pan and sweat the onion rings in it for 8-10 minutes. Then take the pan off the hotplate and let the onions cool down a little.
3. Whisk the eggs with the milk and mix in the onion rings, grated cheese and diced ham. Then add the flour and season the mixture with salt, pepper and the caraway seeds.

4. Pour the mixture into the greased springform pan and bake the onion cake in the oven for 30-40 minutes.

Eggs and spinach nests

Ingredients 4 servings:

- 750 g fresh spinach or frozen
- 4 medium eggs
- salt, pepper

Preparation:

1. Preheat the oven to 175 ° C with a fan oven.
2. Meanwhile, wash the spinach and cook it in boiling and salted water for 2 minutes. Then let it drain and cool before you chop it up and season with salt and pepper.
3. Put the spinach in a baking dish and distribute it well. Make small indentations and slide one egg in at a time. Season the eggs with salt and pepper and put the pan in the oven for 15-20 minutes. When the eggs are set, you can take the baking dish out of the oven and serve the dish on plates.

Italian ratatouille

<u>Ingredients 4 servings:</u>

- 2 medium onions
- 1 medium zucchini
- 1 medium bell pepper, yellow
- 1 medium bell pepper, red
- 1 medium eggplant
- 3 medium tomatoes
- 3 cloves of garlic
- 10 teaspoons of olive oil
- ½ bunch of parsley
- 1 sprig of thyme
- salt, pepper

<u>Preparation:</u>

1. Preheat the oven to 180 ° C fan-assisted.
2. Heat the oil in a small Dutch oven or large saucepan. In the meantime, peel the onion, cut it very small and sweat it in the pot for 5-6 minutes.
3. Then you have to wash the peppers, remove the seeds inside and dice them together with the washed zucchini and eggplant. Then first add the peppers and then the aubergine and zucchini to the pot.

4. Skin the garlic and press it into the pot. Put the sprig of thyme in it and sprinkle everything with the chopped parsley. Then wash all the tomatoes, cut them into quarters with a knife and add them to the other ingredients in the pot. Season the ratatouille with salt and pepper.
5. Then let the stockpot boil down in the oven for 25-30 minutes with the lid closed.
6. Then sprinkle the ratatouille with a little parsley and serve.

Mushroom omelette

<u>Ingredients 4 servings:</u>

- 200 g mushrooms, fresh
- 8 eggs
- 5 tbsp milk
- 2 teaspoons of turmeric paste
- Paprika powder, noble sweet
- 6 stalks of coriander
- 2 tbsp olive oil

<u>Preparation:</u>

1. Preheat the oven to 200 ° C fan oven or 220 ° C electric stove.
2. Clean the mushrooms and chop them into large pieces. Whisk the milk with the eggs, turmeric paste, 1 teaspoon paprika powder and a little salt. Wash the cilantro, shake it dry, and chop the leaves. Stir ¾ of it into the eggmilk mixture.
3. Heat the olive oil in a pan and fry the mushrooms on a high temperature for 2 minutes, turning them over and over again. Pour in the egg-milk mixture and sauté them all again for 3 minutes at medium temperature.

4. Then place the pan in the oven and let the omelette cook there for another 3-5 minutes, until the egg has hardened. Sprinkle the rest of the cilantro on the omelette before serving.

Fish dishes
Crunchy salmon fish fingers

<u>Ingredients 12 fish fingers:</u>

- 500 g salmon fillet, fresh
- 6 tbsp almonds, ground
- 100 g almonds, whole
- 4 teaspoons paprika powder, noble sweet
- 2 teaspoons of turmeric
- 1 teaspoon of ras el hanout
- 6 tbsp olive oil
- salt, pepper

<u>Preparation:</u>

1. Preheat your oven to 200 ° C top / bottom heat.
2. Rinse the fish well under running water and pat it dry. Cut the skin off with a sharp knife, then divide it into 12 equal pieces. Spread the olive oil over the fish and mix the pieces together. Season everything with a little salt and pepper.
3. Put the whole almonds in a blender and chop them into crumbs. Then mix them with the ground almonds, paprika powder, Ras el Hanout and turmeric.

4. Turn the fish pieces one after the other in the breading and then place them on a baking sheet that you have previously lined with baking paper. Now the fish fingers have to bake in the oven for 15 minutes.

5. Serve with the chopsticks an herb quark or other dip to taste.

Teriyaki salmon with leek vegetables

Ingredients 4 servings:

- 8 tbsp soy sauce, without sugar
- 8 tablespoons of tomato ketchup, without sugar
- 4 teaspoons of rice vinegar
- 4 tbsp birch sugar
- 4 cloves of garlic
- 800 g of salmon fillet
- 4 tbsp peanut oil
- 800 g leeks
- 1 small chilli pepper

Preparation:

1. Skin the garlic cloves and squeeze them into a bowl. Mix the soy sauce, ketchup, rice vinegar, birch sugar, and garlic into a sauce. Then put the fish in it and marinate it for 30 minutes.
2. Meanwhile, wash the leek and chilli pepper and cut both into rings.
3. Heat the peanut oil in a pan and fry the leek for 10 minutes. Keep adding a little water to keep it from burning.
4. Then you add the fish to the pan and fry it for 4 minutes.

5. Serve the salmon and leek vegetables on plates.

Fiery lime and salmon fillet from the tray

<u>Ingredients 4 servings:</u>

- 4 salmon fillets
- 1 lime
- 1 red pepper
- 1 green pepper
- 1 bell pepper, yellow
- 1 onion
- 2 tbsp vegetable oil

Marinade:

- 2 limes
- 2 tbsp olive oil
- 2 tbsp water
- 4 cloves of garlic
- 1 teaspoon of cumin
- 1 ½ teaspoon salt
- 1 tbsp honey

- 1 ½ tsp chilli flakes
- ½ bunch of parsley

Preparation:

1. First you have to preheat the oven to 200 ° C and grease the baking sheet with the vegetable oil.
2. Skin the garlic and chop it up. Squeeze out the juice of the limes. Wash the parsley and cut it very small. Mix it with all the other ingredients to make a dressing and set it aside for now.
3. Wash the peppers, remove the seeds, and peel the onion. Cut the peppers into cubes and the onion into rings.
4. Place the salmon fillets on the baking sheet and spread the onions and diced peppers on top. Pour half of the dressing over everything and place the tray in the preheated oven for 10 minutes.
5. Meanwhile, cut the lime into slices. Take the baking sheet out of the oven and spread the remaining dressing over the fish and vegetables. Garnish the dish with the lime wedges and serve.

Salmon and spinach crepes

<u>Ingredients 4 servings:</u>

Crepes:

- 8 eggs, large
- 4 handfuls of spinach leaves
- ½ teaspoon salt
- 4 teaspoons of vegetable oil

Filling:

- 400 g of cream cheese
- 16 leaves of lettuce
- 2 avocados
- 1 cucumber
- 300 g smoked salmon slices
- 1 lemon
- salt, pepper

<u>Preparation:</u>

1. Put the spinach, eggs and ½ teaspoon salt in a blender and mix the ingredients until you have a creamy and green mixture. Let the dough stand for 10 minutes.
2. Heat the oil in a non-stick pan and add a quarter of the batter. Let it set on a low temperature for 4 minutes.

Carefully turn the crepe with a spatula and fry the other side for 1 minute. Repeat this process with the remaining batter until you have at least 4 pancakes.

3. Spread the crepes on plates. Then wash the lettuce leaves, divide the avocados in the middle and remove the stone. Cut the pulp into thin slices. Remove the peel from the cucumber and cut it into slices as well. Squeeze out the lemon juice.

4. Carefully brush the cream cheese over the crepes and place the lettuce leaves on top. Spread some cucumber slices in the middle and cover them with the avocado slices.

5. Then drizzle the lemon juice over the crepes and season with salt and pepper. Spread the salmon on top and carefully roll up the crepes. Finally, cut them diagonally and serve them.

Crab pan with cauliflower

<u>Ingredients 4 servings:</u>

- 1 kg of cauliflower
- 100 g of onions
- 175 g of carrots
- 125 g spring onions
- 250 g of North Sea shrimps
- 5 eggs
- 50 g butter

<u>Preparation:</u>

1. Wash the cauliflower and roughly grate it. Skin the onions and chop them up. Peel the carrots, cut them into cubes and, after washing, cut the spring onions into rings.
2. Heat the butter in a pan and steam the onions in it until translucent. Add the cauliflower and carrots and sauté the vegetables for 7-8 minutes until they are firm to the bite.
3. Stir in the crabs and spring onions. Whisk the eggs and season with salt and pepper. Pour the egg mixture into the pan and let it set. Keep stirring until you have scrambled eggs. Season it with salt and pepper.
4. Serve the crab pan.

Fish with potato wedges

<u>Ingredients 4 servings:</u>

- 500 g white fish fillet, e.g. B. Pollack
- 2 eggs
- 40 g psyllium husks
- salt, pepper
- Paprika powder, noble sweet
- curry powder
- 50 g coconut oil
- 1.2 kg turnip or kohlrabi
- 25 ml of olive oil
- 150 g of Greek yogurt
- 25 g pickles
- 35 g onion, red
- 1 teaspoon mustard, medium hot
- 1 teaspoon balsamic vinegar, light
- 1 teaspoon capers
- 10 g of anchovies in oil

<u>Preparation:</u>

1. Preheat your oven to 185 ° C fan-assisted air.
2. Peel the turnips, cut them into long sticks that look like french fries and pre-cook them in a saucepan for 10 minutes. Then

drain the water and let it drain off. Then spread them out in a large ovenproof dish.

3. Mix the fries with a little olive oil and season them with salt, pepper, paprika powder and curry. Then the fries have to be in the oven for another 20 minutes.

4. Whisk the eggs and season with salt and pepper. Pull the fish through the egg mass and turn it in the psyllium husks. 5. Cut the pickles into small cubes and peel the onion. Then cut the onion very finely. Chop the capers and anchovies.

6. Mix the yogurt with the pickles, onions, mustard, balsamic vinegar, finely chopped capers and anchovies. Season the sauce with salt and pepper.

7. Heat the coconut oil in a pan and fry the fish until crispy.

8. Serve the fish with the sauce and fries.

Redfish in a crispy almond crust

Ingredients 4 servings:

- 8 small redfish fillets or 4 large ones
- 200 g almonds, ground
- 200 g parmesan, grated
- 4-8 eggs, depending on the size
- 100 g almond flour
- 2 lemons
- Chilli flakes
- rosemary
- salt, pepper
- some oil

Preparation:

1. Thaw the fish and then gently pat it dry with a kitchen towel. Cut the rosemary very finely and mix it with the ground almonds and grated Parmesan.
2. Beat the eggs in a tall vessel and whisk them with a little salt, pepper, the chilli flakes and a little lemon juice.
3. Spread the almond flour on a flat plate and toss the fish in it until it's covered all over with the flour. Then turn it in the egg mixture and press the breading firmly.

4. Heat a little oil in a pan and carefully fry the fish fillets until the breading has turned golden brown.

Salmon and cucumber rolls

Ingredients 12 rolls:

- 1 cucumber
- 200 g of cream cheese
- 200 g of smoked salmon
- ½ bunch of dill
- some toothpicks

Preparation:

1. Wash the cucumber, cut off the ends and peel off thin and long slices with a peeler. Place them on a piece of kitchen paper and pat them dry well.
2. After washing, chop the dill and cut the smoked salmon
3. into strips. Brush the long cucumber slices with 1-2 teaspoons of cream cheese, sprinkle some dill over them and place the salmon on top.
4. Then roll up the slices from the side and pin them with a toothpick.

Crispy fish fritters with coconut and zucchini

<u>Ingredients 4 servings:</u>

- 500 g fish fillet, saithe or pangasius
- 2 eggs
- 60 g desiccated coconut
- salt, pepper
- Tarragon, dried
- 2 tbsp chickpeas, ground
- 120 g of cream cheese
- some coconut oil
- 600 g zucchini
- 200 ml coconut milk
- some herb salt
- 1 tbsp parsley, fresh
- 4 tomatoes

<u>Preparation:</u>

1. If you're not using fresh fish, let the fish thaw and cut it into small pieces.
2. Put the eggs, desiccated coconut, fish, salt, pepper, and ground chickpeas in a blender and chop everything up. Taste the mass with the spices again.
3. Heat some coconut oil in a pan and distribute 1 tablespoon of the batter in

each. Fry the pancakes on both sides for 3-4 minutes until golden brown.

4. Meanwhile, wash the zucchini and cut them into small pieces. Heat the coconut milk in a saucepan, place the zucchini in it and cook it for about 10 minutes until it is firm to the bite. Season them with herb salt and pepper. 5. Meanwhile, wash the tomatoes and cut them into slices.

5. Spread the buffers on plates, serve the zucchini vegetables next to them, sprinkle everything with a little parsley and cover everything with 1 slice of tomato.

Cod fillet in mustard crust

<u>Ingredients 4 servings:</u>

- 150 g of lettuce
- 2 tbsp mustard, medium hot
- 1 teaspoon lemon juice
- 2 tbsp balsamic vinegar, light
- 4 tbsp rapeseed oil
- salt, pepper
- 750 g of cod fillet
- 2 eggs
- 5 tbsp flour
- 100 g breadcrumbs

<u>Preparation:</u>

1. Wash the lettuce and gently shake it dry. Mix 1 tablespoon of mustard, lemon juice and balsamic vinegar together and beat in 2 tablespoons of the rapeseed oil. Season the dressing with salt and pepper and fold it into the salad.
2. Rinse the fish under running water, gently pat it dry, and cut it into four pieces. Sprinkle the fillets with a little salt and pepper. Then whisk the eggs with the rest of the mustard. Then turn the fish first in the flour and then

in the mustard-egg mixture and breadcrumbs.

3. Heat 2 tablespoons of rapeseed oil in a pan and fry the fillets for 4 minutes on each side. Arrange the salad and fish on plates and serve.

Fish lasagna with zucchini

Ingredients 4 servings:

- 2 zucchini
- 4 carrots
- 2 cans of chunky tomatoes
- tomato paste
- 2 tbsp cream cheese
- 2 cans of tuna, in its own juice
- 800 g salmon or pollack fillet
- salt, pepper
- garlic powder
- 2 cloves of garlic
- 200 g of feta cheese
- some grated mozzarella
- some marjoram

Preparation:

1. Preheat the oven to 180 ° C fan-assisted.
2. Wash the zucchini and peel the carrots. Cut both into long strips and spread them out on kitchen paper. Sprinkle the vegetables with a little salt to remove the liquid.
3. Skin the garlic cloves and cut them into thin slices. Dice the feta cheese.

4. Sprinkle the fish with a little salt and pepper and fry it on both sides in a pan with a little hot oil. Then add the garlic to the pan and sauté it briefly. Pour the tomatoes over the fish and try to cut up the fish fillets with a spatula to give them a mince-like consistency.

5. Drain the tuna well and add it to the pan. Chop it up a bit too. Season the mixture with salt, pepper, garlic powder and a little marjoram. Then stir in the tomato paste and let the sauce simmer at low temperature for a few minutes. As soon as a creamy sauce is created, you have to stir in the cream cheese and distribute it well in the pan. If it is still too runny, add a little more tomato paste.

6. Now pat the carrots and zucchini dry with kitchen paper and lay them out in a baking dish like lasagne sheets. Spread the carrot strips over it like a grid. This is followed by a layer with the sauce. Spread some crumbled feta on top. Then you have to spread another layer of zucchini and carrot strips in the baking dish, pour the sauce over it and sprinkle with feta. 7. Finally, spread the grated mozzarella over the lasagna and put it in the oven for 20 minutes.

Coconut fish pan

<u>Ingredients 4 servings:</u>

- 1 kg of fish fillet, pangasius or saithe
- 2 zucchini
- 4 peppers, yellow and red
- 2 medium onions
- 200 g broccoli
- 4 spring onions
- 800 ml coconut milk
- 2 pinches of ground ginger
- 2 tbsp rapeseed oil
- 2 tbsp sesame oil
- salt, pepper
- garlic powder
- dill

<u>Preparation:</u>

1. If you're using frozen fish, let it thaw, drain well, and pat it dry. Cut the fillets into bite-sized pieces and season with salt and pepper.
2. Mix the oils together. Wash the zucchini and peppers and cut the peppers into cubes and the zucchini into semicircles. Skin the onion and

chop it up. Divide the broccoli into florets and cut the spring onions into thin rings. 3. Heat the oil mixture in a pan and fry all vegetables except the broccoli in it. Season it with salt, pepper, the garlic powder and a little dill.

3. As soon as the vegetables are well seared, pour in the coconut milk and let it boil briefly. The fish pan should now simmer gently for 15 minutes. When the liquid has reduced a little, you have to add the broccoli. Season with a pinch of ginger.

4. Then put the fish fillets in the pan and let everything boil again briefly. Now the fish pan has to simmer gently for another 5 minutes until the fish is cooked through.

Small coconut balls

<u>Ingredients 20 pieces:</u>

- 250 g cream cheese, low in fat
- 20 g coconut flour
- 30 g almond flour
- 25 g birch sugar
- 3 drops of vanilla flavor
- 20 g coconut flakes

<u>Preparation:</u>

1. Put the cream cheese, the vanilla flavor, the coconut flour, the birch sugar, the almond flour and 10 g coconut flakes in a bowl and mix everything together well until you have a thick mixture.
2. Transfer the remaining coconut flakes to another bowl. Shape the dough into small balls and roll them in the coconut flakes until the entire ball is covered.
3. Place the balls on a plate and then place them in the refrigerator for at least an hour before they can be eaten.

Baked oat flakes with plums

<u>Ingredients 1 serving:</u>

- 5 plums
- 1 egg, organic
- 100 g of Greek yogurt
- 50 g birch sugar
- 1 pinch of cinnamon
- 3 tbsp water
- 40 g of oatmeal
- 1 tbsp peanut butter, unsweetened

<u>Preparation:</u>

1. Beat the egg in a bowl and mix it with the yogurt and 40g birch sugar. Then wash the plums and cut them into pieces. Mix them in with the batter.
2. Grease a round baking pan and pour the batter into it.
3. Turn on the oven and set it to 180 ° C fan oven.
4. Then mix 10 g birch sugar, the pinch of cinnamon, the water, the oatmeal and the peanut butter to a crumbly mass. Spread them on the dough and then put the mold in the oven for 20 minutes.

Fruity lemon cream

Ingredients 4 servings:

- 300 ml lemon juice, fresh
- grated lemon peel
- 6 eggs
- 300 g birch sugar
- 2 teaspoons of cornstarch
- 130 g butter or margarine

Preparation:

1. Put the lemon juice, lemon peel, birch sugar, eggs and cornstarch in a saucepan and stir everything together well. Then place it on the stove and heat the mixture for 10 minutes. Set it to a low temperature. Be careful not to let the contents of the pot start to boil. Keep stirring well.
2. As soon as the lemon mass has a pudding-like consistency, you can take the pot off the stove and let it cool for 5 minutes.
3. Then stir in the butter until it is dissolved. Finally, pour the lemon cream into small glasses and bowls while it is hot.

Pear cake

Ingredients 1 cake:

- 6 eggs
- 300 g birch sugar
- 400 g low-fat quark
- 200 g almond flour
- 2 teaspoons of cinnamon
- 100 g almonds, ground
- 6 pears

Preparation:

1. Preheat the oven to 180 ° C fan-assisted.
2. Beat the eggs and put them in a blender with the birch sugar. Keep stirring until a foamy mass is formed.
3. Mix the quark with the egg mixture and then add the almond flour, ground almonds and cinnamon. Mix the ingredients well together.
4. Grease a round springform pan and pour the batter into it. 5. Wash the pears, cut them in half, remove the core and cut them into slices. Then spread the pear slices on the dough.
6. Put the mold in the oven for 40 minutes.

Summer cottage cheese casserole with berries

<u>Ingredients 1 casserole:</u>

- 500 g low-fat quark
- 50 g cornstarch
- 120 g birch sugar
- grated lemon peel
- 4 eggs
- 12 egg whites
- 400 g raspberries, frozen

<u>Preparation:</u>

1. Put the quark, cornstarch, birch sugar, lemon peel and 4 eggs in a bowl and stir everything together to form a smooth batter.
2. Then beat the 12 egg whites until stiff and fold them into the dough. Then stir in the frozen raspberries.
3. Grease a baking dish and pour the batter into it. Then put the casserole in the oven and let it bake for 15 minutes at 180 ° C hot air until it has turned golden brown.

Rhubarb curd casserole

<u>Ingredients 4 servings:</u>

- 250 ml of milk
- 50 g of semolina
- 15 g vanilla pudding powder, without sugar
- 3 eggs
- 250 g low-fat quark
- 70-80 g birch sugar
- 300 g of rhubarb
- 50 g almond sticks

<u>Preparation:</u>

1. Pour the milk into a saucepan and heat it up. Meanwhile, mix the semolina with the custard powder. Just before the milk boils, you have to stir the semolina and pudding powder mixture into the milk with a whisk. Then take the pot off the hotplate.

2. Separate the eggs and whip the egg whites until stiff. You have to put the egg yolks with the quark, the birch sugar and the semolina-milk mixture in a bowl and stir well until it becomes smooth. Then carefully fold in the egg whites.

3. Now preheat the oven to 170 ° C fan-assisted air.

4. Wash the rhubarb and cut it into pieces. Then grease a baking dish and distribute half of the quark mixture in it. Top the mixture with half of the rhubarb and sprinkle the almond sticks on top. This is followed by another layer with the rest of the quark mass. The remaining pieces of rhubarb are distributed on top and sprinkled with the remaining almond sticks.

5. Place the casserole in the middle of the oven for 35-45 minutes. It tastes best when you serve it warm.

Bundt cake with poppy seeds

<u>Ingredients 1 cake:</u>

- 180 g butter, soft
- 180 g birch sugar
- 6 eggs
- 100 g nuts, grated
- 100 g poppy seeds, grated
- 2 tbsp corn starch

<u>Preparation:</u>

1. Separate the eggs and beat the 6 egg yolks with the soft butter and 140 g birch sugar until frothy. Mix in the poppy seeds, nuts and starch and stir the ingredients well.
2. Beat the egg white until stiff and then let the remaining birch sugar trickle in slowly. Keep hitting until it has dissolved. Then fold the egg white into the batter.
3. Grease a bundt pan, sprinkle some grated nuts into it and fill in the batter. Now the cake has to bake for 1 hour at 160 ° C top / bottom heat in the oven. Then take it out of the oven, let it cool, and then topple it out of the mold.

Carrot pie

<u>Ingredients 1 cake:</u>

- 300 g of carrots
- 5 eggs
- 200 g birch sugar
- ½ teaspoon vanilla, ground
- 300 g almonds, ground
- ½ teaspoon cinnamon
- 3 tbsp lemon juice
- 40 g of finely ground birch sugar

<u>Preparation:</u>

1. Peel the carrots and grate them finely. Separate the eggs and beat the egg yolks with the birch sugar and vanilla powder until frothy.
2. Put the egg whites in another bowl and beat until stiff.
3. Add the carrots, almonds and cinnamon to the egg yolk mixture and carefully fold in the stiff egg white.
4. Grease a springform pan and pour the batter into it. The cake must then bake in the oven at 200 ° C for 35-45 minutes.
5. Meanwhile, prepare the glaze by mixing the lemon juice with the ground birch sugar until a smooth cream is formed. 6.

Take the pan out of the oven, let the cake cool, and turn it out onto a cake plate. When it has cooled down completely, you can coat it with the glaze.

Sugar-free marble cake

<u>Ingredients 1 cake:</u>

- 230 g birch sugar
- 1 pinch of salt
- 1 vanilla pod
- 250 g butter, soft
- 4 eggs
- 160 ml of milk
- 75 g coconut flour
- 425 g almond flour
- 1 packet of baking powder
- 40 g cocoa, unsweetened
- 50 g hazelnuts, grated
- 8 tbsp milk

<u>Preparation:</u>

1. First you have to preheat the oven to 180 ° C top / bottom heat and grease a bundt pan. Then sprinkle in some almond flour.
2. Mix 150 g birch sugar with the salt, the pulp of the vanilla pod and the butter to a creamy mass. Then add 160 ml of milk and the eggs and stir them in.
3. Mix the coconut flour, the almond flour and the baking powder together

and mix everything with the dough mixture to form a smooth dough.

4. Pour half of the batter into the baking pan and stir in 80 g of birch sugar, the baking cocoa, the grated hazelnuts and the 8 tablespoons of milk into the other half. Then fill it into the mold and carefully mix the dough with a fork to create the famous spirals.

5. Place the cake at the bottom of the hot oven and let it bake for 50 minutes.

6. Then let it cool a little in the tin, turn it onto a wire rack and wait until it has cooled down completely.

7. If you want, you can decorate the cake with melted sugar free chocolate.

Ingredients 1 cake:

Ground:

- 90 g butter
- 100 g almonds, sliced
- 100 g almonds, ground
- 65 g almond flour

Filling:

- 250 g of quark
- 750 g of cream cheese
- 80 g birch sugar
- 1 vanilla pod
- 1 vanilla pod
- 1 pinch of salt
- 5 eggs
- 25 g almond or coconut flour
- 200 g strawberries, fresh

Preparation:

1. To start, preheat the oven to 150 ° C top / bottom heat and line a springform pan with baking paper.
2. Then you bring the butter to melt and then mix it with the sliced almonds

and with the ground almonds. Press the batter to the bottom of the baking pan and set it aside.

3. For the filling, mix the quark with the cream cheese and add the pulp of the vanilla pod, the birch sugar and the salt. Then stir in the eggs and almond flour and distribute the mixture on the bottom of the baking pan.

4. Place the cake in the lower part of the oven and let it bake for 1 hour. Then turn off the oven. The cake must then rest for another 30 minutes in the oven, which is still warm. Then place it on a wire rack and let the cheesecake cool down.

Crunchy apple pie

Ingredients 1 cake:

Dough:

- 250 g butter, soft
- 250 g birch sugar
- 1 vanilla pod
- 6 eggs
- 250 g almond flour
- 2 teaspoons of baking powder
- 600 g apple, sour

Covering:

- 100 g almonds, sliced
- 100 g birch sugar
- 100 g butter

Preparation:

1. Preheat the oven to 180 ° C top / bottom heat and line a baking sheet with baking paper.
2. Remove the peel from the apples, cut out the core and cut them into thin slices. Mix the softened butter with the 125 g birch sugar and the pulp of the vanilla pod until frothy. Then add the eggs piece by piece and stir them in.

Mix the remaining flour with the baking powder and mix it with the batter. Then you have to fold in the apple slices.

3. Spread the batter on the baking sheet and bake the cake in the middle of the oven for 30 minutes.
4. In the meantime, heat the butter, birch sugar and almonds for the topping in a saucepan and wait until the butter has melted.
5. Take the cake out of the oven and carefully spread the topping on it. Then the apple pie has to be put in the oven again for 15-20 minutes, until the almonds are baked golden brown. Let the cake cool on a wire rack before serving.

Fruity strawberry Swiss roll

Ingredients 1 Swiss roll:

Biscuit:

- 8 eggs
- 100 g almond flour
- 110 g birch sugar
- 2 teaspoons of baking powder
- ½ vanilla pod

Filling:

- 500 ml of cream
- 2 packets of cream stabilizer
- 300 g strawberries, fresh
- ½ vanilla pod

Preparation:

1. At the beginning, preheat the oven to 160 ° C and cover a baking sheet with baking paper.
2. Beat the eggs with the birch sugar until frothy. Scrape out the pulp of half the vanilla pod. Add the almond flour, vanilla pulp and baking powder to the egg mixture and stir everything well until a batter is formed.

3. Spread the mixture on the baking sheet and bake the dough in the middle of the oven for 12-15 minutes.
4. Then turn the sponge dough out onto a damp cloth and carefully pull down the paper. Roll up the dough with the towel and let it cool.
5. Wash the strawberries and cut them into quarters. Scrape out the pulp of the remaining vanilla pod. Beat the cream, the cream stabilizer and the vanilla pulp until stiff.
6. Roll out the sponge cake and spread the cream on it. Then spread the strawberry pieces on the cream and carefully roll the dough into a roll. Put the cake in the cold for a while before serving.

Quick cup cake

<u>Ingredients 4 servings:</u>

- 4 eggs
- 65 g of cream
- 170 g of cream yogurt
- 1 vanilla pod
- 150 g almond flour
- 80 g birch sugar
- 100 g blueberries

<u>Preparation:</u>

1. Mix all of the ingredients together in a bowl until you have a smooth batter.
2. Divide the batter into 4 microwave-safe cups and place them in the microwave for 2 minutes at 600 watts.
3. Let the cakes cool down briefly and then turn them out onto a plate. They taste good both warm and cold.

Pancakes

<u>Ingredients 4 servings:</u>

- 120 g almond flour
- 200 g almond or soy milk, unsweetened
- 4 eggs
- 40 g of oil
- 1 teaspoon guar gum
- some birch sugar
- some oil

<u>Preparation:</u>

1. Place all of the ingredients in a bowl or in a food processor and stir to form a batter. Let it rest for 10 minutes.
2. Heat 2-3 tablespoons of oil in a pan. Then always add a ladle of batter and bake the pancakes. Turn them over and let them fry until golden brown on the other side as well.
3. Top the pancakes with your desired topping.

CPSIA information can be obtained
at www.ICGtesting.com
Printed in the USA
LVHW050123160621
690353LV00011B/932